Ketogenic Diet

Introductory Beginner's Guide

By Cathy Wilson
Copyright © 2015

Income Disclaimer

This book contains business strategies, marketing methods and other business advice that, regardless of my own results and experience, may not produce the same results (or any results) for you. I make absolutely no guarantee, expressed or implied, that by following the advice below you will make any money or improve current profits, as there are several factors and variables that come into play regarding any given business.

Primarily, results will depend on the nature of the product or business model, the conditions of the marketplace, the experience of the individual, and situations and elements that are beyond your control.

As with any business endeavor, you assume all risk related to investment and money based on your own discretion and at your own potential expense.

Liability Disclaimer

By reading this book, you assume all risks associated with using the advice given below, with a full understanding that you, solely, are responsible for anything that may occur as a result of putting this information into action in any way, and regardless of your interpretation of the advice.

You further agree that our company cannot be held responsible in any way for the success or failure of your business as a result of the information presented in this book. It is your responsibility to conduct your own due diligence regarding the safe and successful operation of your business if you intend to apply any of our information in any way to your business operations.

Terms of Use

You are given a non-transferable, "personal use" license to this book. You cannot distribute it or share it with other individuals.

Also, there are no resale rights or private label rights granted when purchasing this book. In other words, it's for your own personal use only.

Ketogenic Diet

Introductory Beginner's Guide

By Cathy Wilson

Thank you for downloading my book! I appreciate it and I worked hard researching and writing to provide you with the best book possible. Unfortunately I'm not a famous author **yet**, and I don't have at my disposal, a qualified team of writers, researchers, editors, marketers, etc. to put my book on the map. I do it all myself, with the exception of the cover. and I just want to remind you that I am not perfect and neither is this book. I am a very good writer always looking to improve and welcome any constructive criticisms you have to help me deliver bigger and better each time.

If you gain just one piece of useful information, or even just smile once or twice, then I am content. Time to open your mind, enjoy, and look for what you can gain from my book! Thank you again, and at the end of the book, you will find a link to my website and all my other books.

Happy reading!:)

Table of Contents

Introduction

It's safe to say almost every adult on the planet isn't happy with something about their looks. Maybe you feel your nose is too pointy for your face shape, head's too small for your body, or perhaps your waist is tiny and hips gynormous. We're human and most psychologists would agree we are programmed to want what we don't have. Another feature that seems universal is we want to lose weight and we want it to happen **FAST!**

The fat metabolizing Ketogenic Diet is medically based and is designed to force speedy fat burn, which of course is exactly what most people are looking for. It's a proven fast weight loss technique where specific foods trigger fat stores to be used as energy. This diet has captured attention and people want to know more. Based on plenty of healthy fats, some muscle building lean meat, and very little carbohydrates, the body is directed to utilize fat stores first with fat burn as a result.

A chemical change is triggered in energy burn.

According to author and physiologist Lyle McDonald, this diet was first used for treatment of epilepsy. Essentially, the Ketogenic Diet had a medicinal purpose and from there it transformed to a fast weight loss strategy serving the general public.

This diet is extremely popular in the world of body building, weight training, and in particular with other professional athletes that look to drop fat quickly in accordance to their training schedule. However, everyone from soccer moms and construction workers, to successful business people and good old "John Doe's," are experimenting with this fat-blasting eating style in order to get the lean sexy body they desire fast.

Expectations: This book is not technical and is meant to give you a good open and diverse understanding of the Ketogenic Diet, along with other nutrition and health factors that will help to make better decisions for your good health. This book is a platform to gain knowledge in eating. Ultimately taking the positive from it to help you lose weight, gain energy, and build yourself and your life stronger. You may already know some of this information which is great. If you gain just one positive here to improve your health then we both win.

This introductory book outlines the Ketogenic Diet pros and cons, explains how your body burns fat, gives tips and tricks to blast fat for good, and so much more! You will get excited about practical strategies to help you get lean, energized, and healthier to handle all the twists and turns life throws your way. Information is knowledge and I uncover the power to succeed in losing fat for good. Take it if you want it!

Ketogenic Diet Summary

In basic, this eating strategy is strict in eating lots of high fats, moderate protein, and very little carbohydrates. Originally this diet was used medically to treat severe epilepsy in children.

SUMMATION - The body is forced to use fats for energy instead of carbohydrates. Normally the body takes carbohydrates, breaks them down into glucose, which is transported via the blood and used as the energy source for fuelling the body. The body reacts when carbohydrates aren't readily available forcing the liver to turn fat into fatty acids and ketones. What happens is since the brain can't use glucose for energy, it uses ketones. Ketosis is created, which is increased ketones in the blood, reducing the frequency of seizures in epilesy.

Under medical supervision this therapeutic diet allotted just enough protein for muscle growth and repair, and a calculated number of calories for sufficient growth in children. The ratio of fat intake to carbohydrates and protein combined is 4:1. High carbohydrate foods including bread, pasta, white sugar, vegetables and fruits high in starch are eliminated or drastically cut. Higher fat foods like butter and whipping cream are increased.

This diet was created in the early 1920s and many children that suffer from epileptic seizures and have tried this diet notice improvement. Today it's gaining popularity particularly with celebrities, in part because of the huge social pressures dictating "thin is in." Bodybuilders often opt for the Ketogenic Diet during their "cutting phase," where they need to burn fat quickly before a show.

Understanding how your body works, your weight loss goals, health status, and lifestyle, are all keys to determining whether or not this effective weight loss strategy is best suited for you.

Some issues of safety have arisen, but recognizing it's long since been used on children to treat seizures, concerns are minimized. This diet isn't for everyone, particularly those susceptible to liver and kidney issues because of the excess stress of these organs. However, many people practice ketogenic eating and are thinner for it.

My Thoughts . . .

As with any "diet" or eating strategy it's important you run it past your doctor and consider all aspects before chomping down. No one diet to blast fat quickly works for everyone, simply because we all have a different purpose, expectations, tolerances, preferences, and levels of commitment. That's what this book is all about. It gives you the basics of the Ketogenic Diet so you can decide if it fits you.

Basic Body Fat Burning

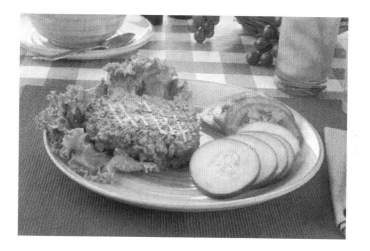

It seems so simple doesn't it? If you just understood how your body burns fat you'd be able to get skinny fast right? Too bad that's not quite how it works. We are all different and this includes metabolizing fat. Physical, mental, social, and emotional factors unique to you will cause your body to burn fat "differently" than everyone else.

Understanding the mechanics behind your metabolism, the rate in which your body breaks down fat, is only going to help you make the necessary changes in your eating and lifestyle to lose weight for good. Let's have a gander at the metabolism to start.

Metabolism

Your digestive system breaks down the foods you eat and transforms them into energy ready for use by your internal systems. The good fats you eat are broken down into fatty acids. Carbohydrates are transformed into glucose ready for use by the brain and internal systems, and amino acids are ready and waiting as an energy source from protein.

Your nervous system, cells and tissues need amino acids and fatty acids to function. Glucose is transported as energy to fuel your body. During carbohydrate use insulin is released to inject the sugars into the required cells. The sugars are then configured into ATP in the mitochondria.

It's a process similar to making gasoline from raw crude oil.

Gaining Fat

Your body needs energy to break food down, for physical activity like hiking and weight lifting, and for intrinsic physiological functioning like blood circulation and your heartbeat. Luckily these are automated or some of us would be in deep trouble. The measurement tool which your body utilizes energy is called your BMR or Basal Metabolic Rate. This represents how many calories your body burns when resting. All but one-third of the energy you use each day is required here. Up to ten percent of the energy you use each day is utilized for the processing of food. This number remains fairly constant always.

When configuring how much you need to eat, it's important to cover your BMR because this is what your body needs to function regardless. If you are exercising and don't want to lose weight, then you will need to factor more food energy into your day so you keep your weight stable. Most often people exercise to burn more energy and lose weight. Theoretically the more you exercise the more fat you will lose, but that's only if you are fuelling your body properly, getting enough lean protein and carbohydrates to build lean muscle and burn fat and you are consistent in eating.

For example, if you are exercising faithfully, but chowing down an extra Big Mac each day, the chances are good you won't lose any weight and likely even add on a few pounds. It case you're wondering, one of these sandwiches has over 600 calories and over half are from fat. A moderate to moderately hard cardiovascular routine will burn about 50 calories per 5 minutes or approximately 300 calories in a half hour. This means to break even you need to get an hour of sweaty cardiovascular activity in. We gain fat by eating more calories than out body needs or uses and it doesn't matter whether they are fat, protein, or carbohydrate calories according to *Men's Fitness*.

The Process

You are continuously burning energy if you are alive. It doesn't matter whether you are water skiing, milking cows, bowling, napping or sipping beverages on the beach, you need energy to do everything.

You lose fat when your intake of energy or food dips consistently below what your body needs or its BMR. This process is cumulative and happens over time. If you eat less calories than your body for just one day and expect to lose weight you will be disappointed. Slow and steady wins the race here.

Take Note: If you starve your body or fall too far below your calories threshold low end your systems will actually stop functioning or at least slow down. This triggers your metabolism to slow and try and conserve energy rather than burn fat. Explaining why people on ultra-low calorie diets can't seem to lose weight no matter how much they exercise and how little they eat.

Bottom line is you have to eat to lose weight!

If you are dieting and aren't giving your body enough nutrients to fuel your systems, naturally your body will break down fat to use for energy. This fat is processed into fatty acids and glycerol. Your muscles, kidneys, and liver use these components and the mitochondria transforms them into ATP. Feels like you're back in biology class doesn't it?

By adjusting the foods you eat and exercising you can communicate to your body to break down more fat for fuel. By weight lifting and building lean muscle you can also help set yourself up for weight loss success. You see muscle naturally burns more calories than fat does. So by transforming your body from flabby to firm and trim you are going to burn more calories at rest or increase your BMR. This means that even when you are having a snooze your body will burn fat!

The foods you eat can also directly affect how much fat you burn or calories expended. The ketogenic diet takes on the initiative of consistently providing less total calories than your body needs to function normally. The result is fat loss and the objective is fast.

My Thinking . . .

We are creatures of habit and if weight loss is the result wanted, then changes need to happen. An open mind and commitment to making eating changes for the better is a must if you want to lose fat. There is no magic pill or concrete strategy that will last long-term in weight loss. If you want to drop 25 pounds and slip back into those sexy skinny jeans you can.

The Ketogenic Diet may be the tool that helps you get healthier fast. Now that you understand how your body uses food and breaks it down fuel and how fat is lost and gained, you can decide whether or not you are ready to the make changes that are going to energize you beyond belief from the inside-out.

Does the Body Need Carbohydrates?

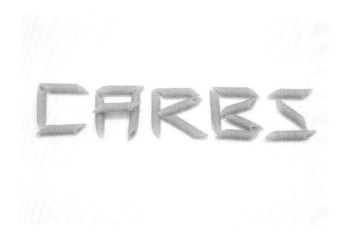

The short answer here is **YES.**

What are Carbohydrates?

Saccharides or carbohydrates are simply sugars and starches that give energy to your body. Many people refer to them as "carbs," and they are often viewed as "fabulous" or "awful." Unfortunately technological advances have changed the way carbohydrates are eaten and not for the better. Processed carbs are directly linked to obesity a wide variety of serious disease. In basic there are two kinds of carbohydrates; **simple** and **complex.**

SIMPLE Carbohydrates in dairy products and fruits are quickly absorbed by the body. Think of this as quick energy. The bad sources of simple carbs are in processed foods like cakes, pastries, cookies, muffins, sweets, white bread, and rice and pasta. Loaded with chemicals and preservatives, it's this simple carbohydrate that will cause interference in your body, trigger weight gain, steal your energy, increase serious disease, and even interfere with thinking.

COMPLEX Carbs have fiber and other important nutrients and take longer to digest. This means you will feel full longer. These good carbohydrates are found in vegetables, whole grain breads, rice and pasta, and beans for example. What type of carbohydrate and how much is where people tend to get into trouble and end up adding fat to their frame. Carbohydrates are used in your body for energy and to help ensure muscle protein isn't used for energy. The last thing you want is for your body to breakdown muscle for energy. Carbohydrates also provide energy for your brain, level blood sugar, and help with muscle recovery after exercise.

The Ketogenic Diet allots for just enough carbohydrate intake for this function.

If you aren't giving your body enough carbohydrates it will automatically use fat and protein for energy but just for a short amount of time. Ketosis is the process in which fat and protein is transformed into energy. This forces ketones to raise in the blood which boosts the acidity of your blood.

Carb Processing

It's your liver that breaks down carbohydrates into simple sugars or glucose for energy. The glucose taps the pancreas which starts up insulin production. Again it's the insulin that has the key that fits the sugars (energy) into the awaiting cells, the type of carbohydrate eaten, simple or complex, good or bad, that dictates how insulin will be produced.

It makes sense that simple sugars are absorbed lickety-split, spiking blood sugar level so you are on an energy high short-term. Grabbing a chocolate bar or soda are unhealthy examples of fast energy that peaks and drops at warp speed. Complex carbohydrate sources take longer to digest and this will result in level blood sugars and long-term energy burn. The insulin result is less.

Some of the excess glycogen from your carb intake can be stored in your muscles and liver cells for small stores of fast energy. It's something athletes are experts in taking advantage of. If however there's too much glycogen it goes directly to your fat stores.

Negative Effects of no Carbohydrates

* extreme fatigue
* cramps in muscles
* poor concentration
* problems thinking

Keep in mind your body can produce energy from fat and protein short term. Even with the Ketogenic Diet some carbohydrates are eventually required.

My Thoughts . . .

You can see that carbohydrates are required for optimal body function, which the Ketogenic Diet allows in small amounts. The focus of this diet is to maximize fat burn by forcing your body to break down fatty acids and amino acids from fat and protein intake for energy. If this is happening, then you're zapping your fat stores. It's a choice and what works for one person may or may not work with another.

Pros and Cons

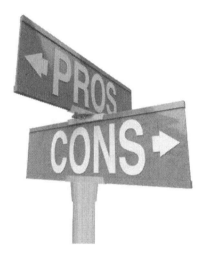

We know ketosis is the process in which your body is forced to burn fats for energy rather than carbohydrates. It is triggered by extremely low carb intake and high fat. As with everything in life there's always the other side of the fence to consider.

VIP - Before attempting any sort of new eating or exercise regimen you should always run it by your medical practitioner just to be safe.

PLUSES

Fat Loss

This is the key focus with the Ketogenic Diet. Studies. They show that ketosis may help you increase the rate in which your body burns fat, but only if you consume less calories than your BMR requires, according to *Prevention Magazine.*

Exercising while using this diet will usually speed up the fat loss process further. In particular if you diversify your exercise regimen using a wide range of interval training exercises, with weights and intense cardiovascular activity.

Decrease in Epileptic Seizures

This diet was originally intended to lower the frequency of seizures in children suffering from epilepsy. Scientists don't know exactly what triggers success here, but they do believe the production of ketones helps control seizures. Fact is, your thinking is usually fuelled by glucose. Hence forcing ketosis and a change in brain chemistry may help minimize seizures, according to *Disease Prevention.*

NEGATIVES

Trouble Sticking with it

The Ketogenic Diet is very restrictive and this makes it a challenge for some to stick with. Many people have trouble eating 4:1 fats to protein or carbs. These restrictions make it harder to adapt in "*the real world,*" because of things like work parties and other social functions, and eating out too. Some people not using this diet to help with seizures will throw in the towel because of the challenge.

Eventual Health Troubles

By eating high-fat foods long term to get your body in a state of ketosis you can trigger long-term health issues. A lot of foods that have higher fat levels are lower in protein and carbohydrates, including lard and coconut oil. Heart disease is increased with a high fat diet according numerous research studies. Evidence also suggests in some instances fats, including more fat than usual, can cause issue with your cognitive capacity over time.

Possible Headaches/Tiredness

The body is used to using glucose for energy so forcing the switch to fat energy can be taxing initially, triggering head pain, unusual tiredness, and even joint pain.

My Thoughts . . .

Understanding both the pros and cons of the Ketogenic Diet is vital in figuring out if it will benefit you. We are each shaped differently. You may be predisposed to headaches and painful migraines which may be enough to steer you clear of this eating strategy. Perhaps you have no issues dealing with a potential mild headache during the adjustment phase when the tradeoff is fast fat loss. That decision is yours to make and the more information the better.

Who Should Follow Ketogenic Diet

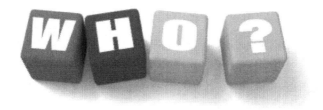

Not everyone should drop everything and adopt to ketogenic eating. Please keep in mind many people following this plan do so under a doctor's supervision, just to be safe. Regardless, any food eating changes you are thinking of executing should be run past your doctor just to be on the safe side.

A tennis player may be someone not suited for this rather strict low-carb eating, mainly because their body is much too dependant on carbohydrates for energy. In other words they have such a high demand from their body for gynormous continuous amounts of energy that ketogenic eating likely just won't work. This doesn't mean they can use this eating style on occasion. It just means it probably isn't a good idea to rely solely on it.

Fact is other people just don't seem to function well overall when carbs are restricted. There's no rhyme or reason that's obvious, it just is. Your body is unique to you and this means it's important you make the choice as to whether or not the Ketogenic Diet is the best choice for you to lose fat fast. You'll only figure this out by trying it in most instances.

There are some scientists claiming harm to liver and kidney function when this low-carb diet is practiced long term. The main reason is because of the high-fat content which can raise blood pressure and cholesterol, stressing the organs considered and system as a whole. Of course you could then look into what kinds of fat these people are eating. That could very well be the culprit.

There's a huge difference between nasty Trans fats and unsaturated healthy fats. Always check with your doctor first. Information is knowledge and it will help you make the best decision for you and your body.

The Ketogenic Diet restricts carbohydrates to less than 50 grams per day, according to *The Mayo Clinic*. That's a huge adjustment for most that likely currently take in ten times that each day.

Sample Breakfast

Here you are looking to have veggies that are non-starch with a maximum 15 grams of carbohydrates. Add to this some protein and fat.

Try…
3 eggs scrambled in olive oil with olives, onions, mushrooms and spinach
Or…

2 eggs cooked in sunflower oil, 2 sausages, 2 slices bacon with sliced tomato

Sample Lunch

This seems to be the time where people gravitate towards eating whole grains, like in a sub or sandwich. You want to avoid these grains, high sugars and fruits for the most part. Often a salad is the easiest for lunch.

Try...
Plate filled with spinach, Romaine, iceberg lettuce, arugula
Add cucumber, avocado, and tomato
Top with a chicken breast, 2-3 hardboiled eggs, steak or salmon steak cooked in olive oil
Toss on some shredded cheese and nut mixture with a low-carbohydrate salad dressing
Or...
6 oz steak grilled in olive oil and onions, wrapped in Romaine, topped with cheese

Sample Dinner

Dinner is easiest with a nice portion of protein and non-starchy veggies. Again ensuring your carbs don't rise about that 15 gram mark.

Try...
A 6-8 oz portion of fish cooked in olive oil
Served with a nice portion of Brussels sprouts and red peppers
Or...

A 6-8 oz serving of chicken, steak or meatballs cooked in olive oil
Add about 2 cups of broccoli or green beans.
It's important between the meat and vegetables that you use 1-2 tbsp of fat.

Sample Snacks

With your snacking you're looking to get less that 5 grams of carbs, plenty of protein and fat.

Try...

1/2 cup cubed cheese

Or...

1/2 cup mixed nuts

Or...

Celery with 2 tbsp natural peanut butter

Or...

1/2 cup tuna on cucumber slices

Or...

2 hard-boiled eggs

My Thoughts . . .

The Ketogenic Diet is quite restrictive in the number of foods you are "allowed" to eat. Although within these groups of food there is huge diversity. So it depends on how you look at it. Is your glass half full or half empty here?

The key factor is to make certain you keep your carbohydrate intake below 50 grams each day. Initially people claim this to be quite the challenge. But as with most things if you stick it out and make it habit you just won't miss it.

Foods Considered Ketogenic

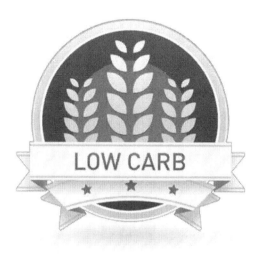

As we've already discovered, Ketogenic eating focuses on protein, high fat, and low carbs for fuel. That said, meat is the basic food substance mainly because meat doesn't have carbs. This is the key signalling your brain to use amino acids and fatty acids for fuel.

Meat - Experts suggest eating a variety of fat and lean meats because too much fat can send your cholesterol levels up.

Fat Cuts
- beef
- pork (shoulder, ribs, belly)
- chicken (dark meat)
- turkey (dark meat)

Lean Meat

- chicken (white meat)
- turkey (white meat)
- beef (sirloin, round, flank, tenderloin)
- pork (tenderloin)

Fish is the best source of ketogenic food because fish options like salmon and sardines are fatty fish which are great sources of omega 3 fatty acids. These keep your heart healthy!

Oil - Oils are also a dominant ketogenic food because they're fat. Prime choices are canola oil, olive oil, and co-conut oil. The first two are considered unsaturated and healthy fats, liquid at room temperature and heart healthy. Coconut oil is one those foods that's slipped be-tween the cracks. Technically it's considered a saturated or unhealthy fat. But research shows this oil is actually excellent for your health.

Not just by helping to regulate and support your internal system function, but also to protect from nasty free radi-cal, clear up skin conditions and leave your hair, nails, and skin boasting healthy, according to Dr. Oz.!

It's used to treat everything from diaper rash to eczema and blemishes. Coconut oil is definitely one exception to the rules and should be included in your healthy eating plan in moderation. Sesame and corn oil are also healthy oils to include in your Ketogenic Diet.

Vegetables - Contrary to what some believe vegetables are part of this diet plan, just not in the capacity you might normally eat. Many, but not all vegetables are high in carbohydrates.

Do Vegetables

* broccoli
* asparagus
* romaine and iceberg lettuce
* spinach
* red, green, orange and yellow peppers
* cucumbers
* olives
* artichokes
* summer squash
* zucchini
* mushrooms
* celery
* turnip greens

Don't Vegetables
* peas
* corn
* potatoes
* carrots

Fruits - Most people think of fruits as high carb and high in sugar and they're right. Although there are some fruits suitable for a rather strict low-carb diet like the Ketogenic Diet.

Olives are excellent along with cranberries, raspberries, blackberries, lemons, and rhubarb. Some of the fruit choices with medium levels of carbs and sugars are peaches, blueberries, oranges, grapefruits, pineapple, watermelon, and apples. Select these only on occasion.

Don't Eat
* bananas
* cherries
* grapes
* dried fruit
* figs

Milk and Milk Products - Most dairy products have little or no carbohydrates so they fit well into the Ketogenic Diet. Having a higher fat content also makes them ideal.

One thing you do need to watch out for is the natural sugars in milk and milk products, like lactose in milk. This just means you should consume these particular food options moderately.

Best Choices
* various cheeses
* sour cream
* natural yogurt

Condiments/Extras - It's very important to have a look at the ingredient list of the condiments or extra toppings before you use them. Many have hidden sugars and carbohydrates that you need to be aware of.

Best Choices
* soy sauce
* mustards
* creamy saucy
* butter sauces

Keep in mind condiments and extras should be used sparingly regardless.

Beverages - The drinks included with this diet are essentially the same as any low-carb eating plan. Stay away from sugar sodas and choosing diet soda if you must.

Picking caffeine-free coffee and tea are smart moves and of course all natural water is the best. Making sure you get 6-8 glasses each day on the lower end. When looking at alcohol, beer, and mixed drinks, they are off limits because of the high sugars and carbohydrates. An occasional "hard liquor" drink is okay in moderation.

These are "empty" calories remember.

My Thoughts . . .

It's fair to say this diet is much more restrictive than most low-carb diets out there. There's give and take with everything and if you want results, fat loss fast, then you'll have to buckle down and adjust.

If not, there are lots of other similar diets out there to explore. Keep at it and eventually you will find gather all the information you need to create and stick with an eating and lifestyle plan that works for you. Most people that use this ketogenic eating style will admit the initial adjustments were psychosomatically and physically taxing.

After they persevered through this "shock" to the mind and body they adjusted nicely and were extremely happy with the results. As always the choice is yours to make with the information you are gathering and processing.

Interesting Nutrition Facts

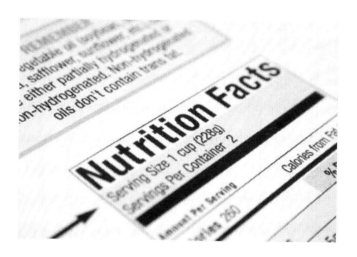

Tips to Prevent Vitamin Loss in Food

Here are a few pointers to help steer clear of losing precious vitamins and minerals in the foods you eat:

*steam your vegetables
*use minimal amounts of water when steaming so nutrients don't seep out
*don't bother defrosting frozen foods before cooking
*keep milk product cool and don't allow any sun exposure because this steals vitamins
*don't soak veggies in water before cooking, just rinse in cool water
*store beans and peas in paper bags to prevent vitamin B2 depletion
*buy fresh always just enough for a few days at a time

*cook in stainless steel to prevent loss of essential vitamins and minerals

What are Proteins?

Proteins are the building blocks of your body. The protein you eat gets broken down into 20 different amino acids, which are used for energy, according to *Science Daily*. If you are eating "complete" protein, usually from an animal source, you will provide your body with all of the AA required for good health.

Most plant sources, with the exception of quinoa, are not complete. This means you need to eat them in combination to provide your body with the complete protein it needs to function optimally.

Proteins help build muscle and maintains cells. They also produce hormones and various other antibodies. The good health of your bones, skin, and hair are dependant on adequate protein.

All Fats Aren't Created Equal

There are good and bad fats, namely unsaturated and saturated respectively. In the "good" fat department you'll find polyunsaturated (omega 3 and 6), the ones your body can't live without. Your brain needs them to function and they help prevent serious cancers and other diseases.

Monounsaturated fats are also good for you, but not essential. They are associated with ensuring your cholesterol levels are within the normal range.

Bad fats that are unsaturated, including synthetic or chemically altered trans-fats that are not required by your body. They build up in your body to toxic levels, create interference in good health, and can cause obesity, diabetes, high blood pressure and cholesterol to start.

You Can't Live Without Water

Most people are aware your body is made up of about 65% water. Losing just 5% of your water capacity can result in serious dehydration issues.

Here are a few important points with regards to pure refreshing water:

*flushes harmful toxins from your body
*lubricates internal systems for better function
*it helps prevent cancers and other serious disease
*carries oxygen through to vital organs and internal systems
*helps to increase weight loss and increase metabolic processes
*improves digestions and helps carry nutrients throughout your body for use
*is necessary for saliva production and keeping joints functioning optimally
*decreases the chances of intestinal issues like constipation

Nutrition is...

The word nutrition is made from "nourish," which is from the Latin word "nutrire," to feed and support. In general nutrition is the way in which the body uses food.

Diseases Caused by Poor Nutrition Are:

*Scurvy (lack of vitamin C)

*Pellagra (lack of B3)
*Anemia (lack of B12)
*Osteomalacia/Rickets (lack of vitamin D, calcium, phosphate)
*Xerophthalmia-blindness from infection (lack of vitamin A)

Vitamin D Fact

Vitamin D is a unique vitamin because it's the only one your body can synthesized. If you are always wearing sunscreen you can block essential vitamin D. This vitamin also holds the title of the only vitamin that's a hormone.

"Vitamin" Termed

Casimir Funk was a chemist that's credited for defining "vitamin." It comes from "vital," which means necessary for life and "amine," a compound that has hydrogen and nitrogen. They were founded starting in 1900 and later scientists figured out all weren't amines.

Temperature Matters

Did you know that cold people in general are more likely to eat more than someone who is warm? Studies show that appetite can be affected by temperature.

Minerals

Calcium, sodium, and iron are minerals that make up about 5% of your body weight. Minerals don't give off energy.

Experts Agree…

The best way to lose weight is to eat less calories and exercise more. The Ketogenic Diet will help you cut calories and lose weight.

Get Cracking

Eggs have the highest quality of protein. And did you know the shell of an egg has lots of calcium?

Easy on the Caffeine

100 cups of coffee in less than 5 hours technically is lethal.

Meat Stamps

The dye used to stamp meat is edible, made from grape skins.

Mushrooms Beware

The Amanita phalloides is termed the death cap. This mushroom contains five different poisons. Most people that eat them end up in a coma and then die.

My Thoughts . . .

There are always going to be little odds and ends to learn about nutrition. Hopefully these enlighten and add to your overall nutritional arsenal, or perhaps just some neat conversation for around the coffee table.

Lightly Science - Cancer and Carbs

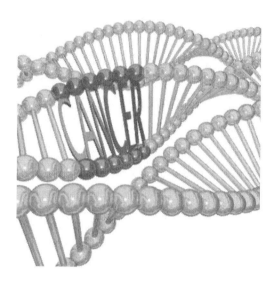

Science seems to have this magical power over the mind. If science says it's true it must be! Regardless, there's always room for error even in science. The procedure could be executed incorrectly, or the results could be fudged. It doesn't seem to matter because so many people take science as fact **NO MATTER WHAT!**

Recently, scientists and medical experts have been reporting consistently that the Ketogenic Diet can actually kill cancer cells, by feeding the body a fat-based diet scientists report the death of cancer cells.

For years experts have agreed that carbohydrates are not good for cancer patients. Most recently Thomas N.

Seyfried, PH.D, suggests normal bodies function fine without carbs, but cancer cells don't. This doctor among others believes a high-fat no carb diet kills all kinds of cancers.

The science behind this, is without dietary sugar cancers cells can't live. There's plenty of research to back this up. Of course there's always some sort of controversy and this theory is no different.

Questions arise as to why patients in stage IV cancer on a high carbohydrate vegetarian diet have success in the battle? One of the many questions researchers are working hard to understand better.

Studies show men have a lifetime risk of 1 in 2 of getting cancer and women 1 in 3, pretty scary stats. In today's world cancer has become an epidemic that shows no signs of slowing anytime soon.

Experts from European countries have reported since the mid 1800s the more grain consumed, the higher risk of cancer. What's proven through science is cancer cells are anaerobic, whereas healthy cells are aerobic. This means cancerous cells don't need oxygen for metabolism.

This has been displayed in Petri dishes where the oxygen was taken away from a healthy cell and it turned cancerous.

The positive is that Dr. David Gregg believes cancer cells can be converted back into healthy cells, aerobic cells, when oxygen and all the minerals and vitamins for aerobic metabolism are present.

He notes in his research these cancerous cells need carbohydrates to divide and grow. They can't use protein or fat. Bottom line is science points to the conclusion a low-carb diet will starve cancer cells. Studies back this concept up showing that cancerous tumors shrink when carbs are removed. This could be just another incredible reason to consider the Ketogenic Diet.

My Thoughts . . .

It's always encouraging to see when a specific eating style does more than boost your overall caloric burn and blast fat. The science behind this diet shows low-carb eating or a no carb diet can actually kill cancerous cells too.

What this does is make the Ketogenic Diet even more useful in the big picture of good health. There are no guarantees in life of course, but these scientific findings really do look promising.

Myths and Truths

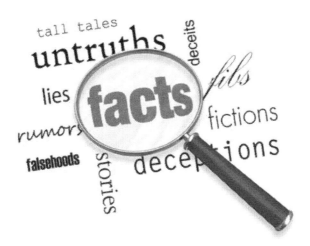

Carbohydrates always seem to be the talk of the diet world. Either getting bashed or gloried, or somewhere in between. Here are a few myths about carbs that just might help you make better decisions for your mind, body, and waistline!

Myth 1 - Fruits and veggies aren't allowed.

Truth - Many believe all fruits and vegetables are mainly carbohydrates, which means they aren't allowed in the Ketogenic Diet plan.

In general if you are eating a low-carb diet you would be choosing vegetables over fruits for the most part. The truth is most people that follow a low-car diet like the Ketogenic Diet, usually eat more vegetables and fruit than the general populous. Eating non-starchy carbohydrates are perfectly fine because are already located on the low end of the carbohydrate scale.

Action - Don't forget the ratio 4:1, fats to protein and carbs. Olives are one of the few fruits that are carbohydrate free. Cranberries, lemons, blackberries, raspberries, and rhubarb are all low in carbs and natural sugars. Veggies including spinach, squash, asparagus, broccoli, cabbage, mushrooms and zucchini also fit.

Myth 2 - Eating a low-carb diet long term will cause kidney problems.

Truth - This is just not true. Truth is low carb diets also have lower protein intake than most "normal" diets. This is good for people suffering from kidney issues.

Myth 3 - Low-carb, high protein diets will cause osteoporosis because of calcium loss.

Truth - First off, the Ketogenic Diet isn't high protein. It is high fat and moderate amounts of protein. Besides that, protein is essential for strong bones according to *The Ontario Beef Council*. Studies show individuals with hip fractures often have inadequate protein intake.

Myth 4 - The only reason you lose weight on a lower carbohydrate diet is because of calorie restriction.

Truth - Simplistically speaking the weight loss occurs on a low carb diet because of a forced change in eating, technicality which gives a metabolic advantage. Think of it as a kick-in-the-butt in your fat burning. It's more about removing excess "empty" calories and replacing them with nutrients and fuel your body needs. It's a re-configuration if you will.

Myth 5 - It's impossible to keep weight off long term with a low carb diet.

Truth - Fact is many people use low carbohydrate eating as permanent fixture in their life. Experts agree it does work for some. Bottom line is you can keep weight off while sustaining a low-carb diet for as long as you choose if you're smart about it.

Myth 6 - Controlled carbohydrate diets like the Kenogenic Diet will increase the risk of heart disease.

Truth - The opposite rings true. Studies show these diets actually decrease markers for heart disease risk. This includes lowering blood fat and blood pressure, as well increasing good cholesterol or HDL. Research at Stanford shows on more than one occasion diets with low carb had better outcomes related to cardiac markers than diets with low-fat, high-carbohydrates.

Myth 7 - The Ketogenic Diet won't help you lose weight. It just causes muscle and water loss.

Truth - These statements are false. What happens is low-carb diets actually form chemical changes in the body promoting fat loss. Numerous studies have been conducted resulting in more fat loss than lean muscle mass compared to other higher carb eating plans.

My Thoughts . . .

Rumors do cause a whole lot of negative interference with good health. If you don't have accurate information to start it's going to be pretty tough for you to reach your weight loss goals. When it comes to carbohydrates, it

seems society views in the extreme. People either be-
lieve they can be part of a healthy diet to lose weight or
they don't. Of course they can and are, but there are a
whole whack of strings attached, depending on your
goals, preferences, tolerances, immediate health and
general knowledge and lifestyle.

Move forward with an open mind and trust your gut. This
will only help you sift through the rocks and find the dia-
monds you need to make the best decisions for you and
your long-term sustainable health.

Ketogenic?Atkins?

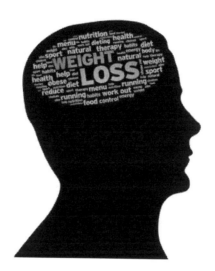

Both the Adkins and Ketogenic Diet plans claim success in weight loss. There are many that find the Adkins Diet more easily sustainable longer term because it's a little more relaxed. By first understanding the basics of both, we can effectively uncover the differences and importance of both styles of eating. What might work for you may or may not work for your neighbor.

Atkins Diet - Officially this diet is referred to as the "Atkins Nutritional Approach" diet that's low-carb based. It's actually supported by researcher Robert Atkins and based on a medical paper he read on weight loss. His approach to weight loss is personal as he used the Atkins Diet to lose weight himself.

The idea with this eating strategy is to force the body to switch fat burning components by reducing the carbohydrates available for energy burn. This forces ketosis, where instead of readily available glucose for fuel the body must now use protein and fat stores for energy.

Without getting to technical here, ketosis is triggered when insulin levels are too low. In general insulin levels are only low when there isn't very much glucose in the body, just before you are about to eat, for example.

Science proves low insulin levels triggers lipolysis and this means fat gets burned instead. The products of this fat burn are ketones or ketone bodies. That's the long and the short of it. Bottom line is more calories are burned because it takes more calories to both make and burn fat.

Ketogenic Diet - This diet is the first level of the Atkins Diet essentially. The Ketogenic Diet relies specifically on insulin response to your blood glucose. Remembering insulin is the natural response to blood sugar levels that are too high, after eating for example.

Livestrong reports the purpose of glucose is to transport glucose from your blood to the awaiting cells and tissues calling for energy. If it isn't used for immediate energy then it's stored as pesky fat. It's exactly what most of America is trying to get rid of.

With this diet an insulin response doesn't happen because not enough glucose in is the system, increasing your metabolism and burning fat for energy instead. The body is also forced to work harder because extra energy is required to transform any stored fuel to glucose. The body ends up completely reliant on fat and protein breakdown for energy short-term and longer term.

Highlighted Differences

Both of these low-carbohydrate diets are very similar. The expected result is fast fat loss by restricting the availability of glucose for energy burn.

The main difference is the Atkins Diet is less restrictive. So you've got a little more wiggle room. With that said, you may not lose the fat as fast with the Atkins Diet because of this factor.

With the Ketogenic Diet you are aiming to keep carbs below 50 grams per day for maximum effect.

The Atkins Diet doesn't restrict protein, fat, or calories like the Ketogenic Diet does. Which may come in handy for people that are immune to portion control to start.

In my opinion everything has a limitation. It's a line that when crossed takes you over into the negative. The Ketogenic Diet strategy might very well keep you on the "right" side of this line.

My Thinking . . .

This choice comes down to how badly you want to lose fat, your overall health, and preferences and tolerances.

If you are in poor health and can't stand eating restrictions, the Ketogenic Diet plan may not be for you. However if you are training for a bodybuilding show and need to slim down fast, the Ketogenic Diet might work perfectly for you.

What's important is that you first gather as much information as you can and then start with the process of figuring out if you will set yourself up for success committing to the Ketogenic Diet plan or not.

FAQ's

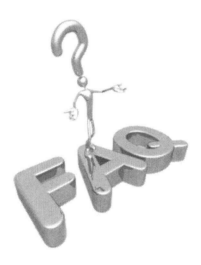

Considering this eating plan is new to you there are always going to be a few questions that still need to be answered. Here are a few Frequently Asked Questions that hopefully will satisfy a few more thoughts you are pondering.

Question One - Can you eat as much as you want and still lose weight if you are restricting carbohydrates?

The answer here is no. By reducing your carbohydrates you are reducing calories but if you over consume in the protein and fat department you aren't going to lose fat, regardless in the new metabolic process being utilized.

The thinking is that carbohydrate intake in our society today is often the source of vast amounts of fat or nutrition-less calories. By essentially getting rid of the factor or eating you are opening up room for more protein and fats in your diet and still lose weight. Although you really can't eat a cow minus the grass and still expect to lose weight.

Question Two - Does the Ketogenic Diet have side effects?

Doesn't pretty much everything you do in life? Some are good and others bad. This answer is unique to each individual because some people notice affects more than others. It's the same as one person may get a paper cut and scream. Another might not even notice it.

The risk for side effects does increase with obese people, namely because most are already predisposed to health conditions affecting their heart and other organs. In other words these individuals are already "damaged."

Question Three - What are a few of the more common side effects?

*dehydration
*ketosis
*calcium depletion
*nausea
*weakness
*electrolyte loss
*kidney and liver issues

There can also be issues with vitamin and minerals. This diet is restrictive and a supplement is recommended to ensure you are getting all the vitamins and minerals your body requires to zap fat and stay healthy.

Question Four - Can you get gout?

On occasion gout is a potential side effect. This is because there's an increase in uric acid because it's in competition with ketone bodies for excretion. High levels of uric acid in the blood can also trigger kidney failure on rare occasion. Just to be safe it's recommended people with kidney issues don't follow this diet unless under close supervision by their doctor.

Question Five - Can you drink alcohol on this diet?

The short answer is yes, but any alcohol does slow the process of fat breakdown. A drink on occasion is allowed but stick to hard liquor and not mixed drinks and beer which are high in carbohydrates.

For example, a whiskey on the rocks or with diet soda would pass. Again, if you are serious about burning fat alcohol really just shouldn't be on your main menu.

Question Six - Will a child on this diet get fat?

Normally a child on this diet is using it to help treat epilepsy and is under strict supervision, which means a child isn't likely to get fat because a nutritionist will make sure the calories allowed won't be in excess of the physical demands of the body. Bottom line is if the total calories are limited, the amount of fat within the diet won't cause weight gain.

Question Seven - Can prescriptions interfere with this diet?

Regardless of whether you are referring to toothpaste, cold medicine or prescriptions, they must all be sugar-free and carbohydrate-free. This means you must check

with both your doctor and pharmacist to make certain you
are complying.

My Thoughts . . .

*These are just a few of the FAQ that might be of interest
to you. As always if you have a question, don't hesitate to
ask your doctor, pharmacist, or other qualified expert.*

The only "dumb" question is the one not asked!

Final Words

Most people seem to be born impatient and are always looking for the golden ticket to fast fat loss. This is why fat diets are a multi-billion dollar industry that just keeps on going and going and going.

Bottom line is the Ketogenic Diet is more or less successful as a whole in weight loss compared to all the others of the scientific/medical community. Where you may run into trouble is with the high fat content that might not help someone who isn't disciplined in the concept of healthy eating. Or someone that doesn't understand moderation and reasonability. Just because this diet is high-fat doesn't mean you get to hit the fast-food outlets. That's not what this is about.

The Ketogenic Diet requires thorough understanding **BEFORE** you begin. One must be in tune with their body and understand at least the basics of what your body needs to survive, burn fat, and stay healthy.

Due to the fact this Ketogenic Diet actually reconfigures your fat burning process. But you need to first be committed to making the changes and then to following through with the blessing of your healthcare provider.

Will you lose fat quickly on this diet plan? Yes, that's pretty much a given.

Can you sustain this eating style and stay healthy? Yes, with an open mind, supervision, and a constant monitoring of your progress.

Don't forget about taking a daily supplement just to be safe.

Is the Ketogenic Diet worth it? Well this answer is up to you. It very well could be if that's what **YOU** choose.

If you gained just one important piece of information to help you make better decisions in your health by reading this book, then I've done my job and am thoroughly pleased for you. That's what this world should be all about, helping each other simply because we can and want to.

We have the choice to look for the positive or the negative in life. You can choose to lift someone up or to stomp on them. Writing is my passion and I work hard at it, with the goal of helping make people better. If you gain a new piece of knowledge, read something that makes you think, or perhaps even smile a few times, then I am happy and content!

Life's just too short not to tune into optimism. If your glass is half full, then I invite you to read my writing, and if you have a minute to spare when you're through, **I would appreciate your review.** This will help me better myself and my writing. I thank you in advance and appreciate you.

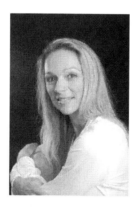

I hope that you enjoyed my book and you can check out all my other books on my website at:
http://www.flawlesscreativewriting.com

Made in the USA
San Bernardino, CA
29 August 2016